L-Lysine and Inflammation

Herpes Virus - Pain - Fatigue - Cancer,
How Do We Control These

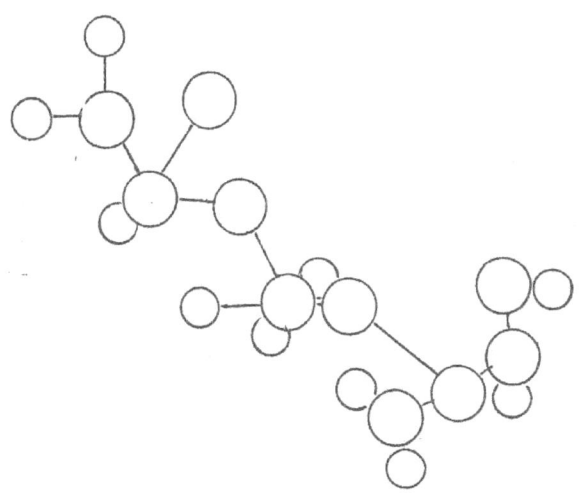

Dr. Robert G. King Jr.

Copyright © 2014 Dr. Robert G. King Jr.
All rights reserved.
ISBN: 1495976548
ISBN 13: 9781495976544
Library of Congress Control Number: 2014903319
CreateSpace Independent Publishing Platform
North Charleston, South Carolina

ACKNOWLEDGMENTS

I wish to give special thanks to Nancy J. Huntington for providing her technical assistance in using the electronic media to produce this book.

My wife, Emily D. King, provided invaluable assistance with suggestions to make this book more understandable to those unfamiliar with medical jargon.

As a member of the medical community for fifty years, I am very fortunate to be part of the the very best medical care system available. This system allows individuals to discuss their experiences and opinions. Hopefully, such information will benefit others.

TABLE OF CONTENTS

INTRODUCTION vii

CHAPTER 1 1

CHAPTER 2 7

CHAPTER 3 13

CHAPTER 4 21

CONCLUSION 27

ABOUT THE AUTHOR 31

INTRODUCTION

The greatest wealth is health ...... Virgil

Most of us take health for granted until we feel it is no longer as good as we would like. In our teens and twenties we seldom are sick except for respiratory infections which either clear on their own or if bacterial, will clear with antibiotic treatment. We can eat high calorie foods with hydrogenated oils and high fructose corn syrup and still feel healthy. Our bodies have a tremendous capacity to clear toxic chemicals and overcome bad habits of reduced exercise and poor hygiene.

In our thirties, modern medicine still keeps us healthy. We have treatment plans to control blood pressure and blood sugar. Antibiotics can clear most bacterial infections and antiviral drugs can control viral infections such as chickenpox and herpes. We also have vaccines for childhood diseases and genital infections such as the papilloma viruses.

As we reach the forties, our immune system is not as effective to fight inflammation. Our focus or accommodation begins to decrease resulting in difficult reading. Our joints begin to wear and deteriorate as we exercise more to try to control weight and increase stamina.

The fifties bring on prostate problems for men and breast problems for women. Diseases such as these present with multiple symptoms and it becomes difficult to differentiate between the inflammation of aging or cancer.

The sixties and seventies are concerned with treatments to maintain general health. There are concerns with which medications are the most effective to maintain good health and not produce side effects. Inflammation of the vascular system needs to be controlled to maintain blood flow to vital organs. Antioxidants are prescribed to maintain retinal health and help prevent retinal macula degeneration. Foods with high phytonutrients need to be included in the diet to reduce free radicals to prevent cellular damage.

The eighties and nineties should have treatment plans in place with attention to new concepts concerning healthy brain function. As more research is performed, it appears that the control of inflammation is the critical factor in good health. Inflammation causes decreased blood flow in vessels and results in damage to body organs such as the brain, eyes, heart and digestive tract.

I have developed the following observations and concepts concerning inflammation as a result of my fifty years of medical practice of Ophthalmology. Hopefully this discussion will lead to a better understanding of inflammation and result in better health.

Dr. Robert G. King Jr.

INTRODUCTION

WORDS for COMPUTER SEARCH

BACTERIA -

VIRUS -

INFLAMMATION -

ANTIOXIDANTS -

L-Lysine and Inflammation

PHYTONUTRIENTS -

FREE RADICALS -

CHAPTER 1

Truth is never pure and rarely simple.... Oscar Wilde

Inflammation in the body is a normal response to injury or some attack by bacteria, viruses or parasites. The body's immune system senses an abnormal situation and can produce redness, swelling, pain and heat. This type of inflammation is usually characterized as acute and results in active treatment to alleviate the situation.

Chronic inflammation can occur at such a low level in the body that very few symptoms are present until the damage becomes severe enough to produce abnormal blood sugar, blood pressure or such blood tests as an elevated c-reactive protein. Many life style situations such as obesity, smoking, sedentary habits, excessive stress and exposure to environmental toxins can produce chronic inflammation.

As an ophthalmologist, I have the advantage of being able to visualize eye inflammation with various instruments and still leave the eye intact. The cornea can become infected with a herpes simplex virus which produces pain, sensitivity to light and possible decreased vision. This condition is called herpetic keratitis and usually clears with treatment; however, it can reoccur and produce corneal scarring. Corneal surgery then is needed to restore useful vision. The diagnosis is made by applying various stains to the front of the cornea. A dendritic or branching pattern is diagnostic of corneal herpes. This diagnosis is made visually and does not require cultures or blood tests. When the cornea no longer stains, the infection is inactive and a decision can be made to terminate the treatment.

I found in the 1960's that a treatment using the essential amino acid supplement L-lysine appeared to decrease the reoccurrence of corneal herpetic infections. The use of L-lysine in this fashion is a complementary medical treatment to make the usual medical treatment more effective.

In 1963, I did not need to use L-lysine as much because of the introduction of a new antiviral drug called 5-iodo-2'-deoxyuridine or IDU. This drug in the form of a eye drop competed with thymidine and other purines in the virus DNA to control the virus. The drug did not kill the virus but it did appear to decrease reoccurrences.

In 1974, an acyclovir drug was approved to treat viral infections. Today we have multiple drugs for eye and systemic viral infections: however, they do not appear to kill the virus since there can be reoccurrences of the disease.

The herpes virus is classified as either type 1 or type 2. Type 1 infections often occur around the mouth and eye areas. Type 2 infections often occur in the genital area. Some other types of viral infections are herpes zoster infections (shingles), chickenpox (varicella), cytomegalovirus,

Dr. Robert G. King Jr.

Epstein-Barr and the human papilloma virus. Some viruses seem only to cause infections while others like the human papilloma virus can cause cancer.

After prescribing L-lysine in the past for herpetic corneal infections and also using this supplement to help clear fever blisters, I would like to discuss in the following chapters my experiences using L-lysine as a supplement to produce a healthier life style with more stamina.

CHAPTER 1

WORDS for COMPUTER SEARCH

HERPETIC KERATITIS -

L-LYSINE -

COMPLEMENTARY MEDICINE -

I D U -

Dr. Robert G. King Jr.

ACYCLOVIR -

CORNEA -

THYMIDINE and PURINES -

CHAPTER 2

Man shall not live by bread alone.....Matthew IV 4

L-lysine is one of ten essential amino acids. The biologic action of L-lysine directly depends on L-arginine which is also an essential amino acid. The amino acid structure of proteins defines it's biological activity and cellular function. Humans can produce ten of the twenty amino acids which make up proteins. Those that can not be produced are called essential amino acids and must be supplied by food intake or supplementation. Amino acids are not stored in the body; therefore, daily ingestion is necessary to avoid amino acid deficiency.

It appears that the amount of L-lysine as compared to the amount of L-arginine in the human body is related to L-lysine's antiviral activity. The greater the amount of L-lysine, it is harder for the viruses to grow. The greater the amount of L-arginine, it is easier for virus to grow. Antiviral activity can be increased by ingesting more L-lysine or by avoiding foods high in L-arginine.

L-Lysine and Inflammation

L-lysine intake can be increased by supplementation but it is best to consume foods high in L-lysine. Some of these foods are red meats, eggs, fish, legumes, brewer's yeast and dairy products such as yogurt and cheese. To decrease the amount of L-arginine consumed, foods such as some vegetables, fruits, nuts, oats and wheat products should be consumed in smaller amounts.

L-lysine supplementation can vary from 500 mg. to 3 grams daily. To treat conditions such as fever blisters, 3 grams can be taken daily for a week if there are no side effects. For long term daily supplementation, 500 mg. is best. As with any ingested substance, attention should be paid to adverse reactions. The most common side effect of L-lysine ingestion is nausea and vomiting.

Anyone who takes L-lysine as a daily supplement should have yearly liver and kidney chemistry profiles done when blood is drawn. L-lysine is metabolized by the liver and excreted by the kidneys.

As with any supplementation or food plan, a physician should be aware of your actions. In addition, pregnancy and lactation require special medical attention.

If an anti-inflammatory lifestyle is the objective, a food plan such as the Mediterranean diet along with supplementation of vitamins, minerals, amino acids and probiotics should be considered. There are many conditions in the body which seem to be associated with inflammation and possibly this type of lifestyle change could be beneficial.

In the next chapter I will outline the food plan I use to decrease inflammation and produce a healthier life style.

CHAPTER 2

WORDS for COMPUTER SEARCH

ESSENTIAL AMINO ACIDS -

L-ARGININE

ANTI-INFLAMMATORY FOODS -

MEDITERRANEAN DIET -

PROBIOTIC -

L-LYSINE TO L-ARGININE RATIO

CHAPTER 3

Let food be your medicine and medicine be your food...Hippocrates

As with any food regimen, it is better to consume essential nutrients in natural form; however, supplements can be used to get more concentrated nutrients if food restrictions are present. As an example, if dairy products and meats cause digestive upset, a L-lysine supplement can be taken.

One of the foods I try to eat is buckwheat. It is a seed which probably was cultivated as early as 6,000 BC in Asia. It has high concentrations of L-lysine and is gluten free. It also contains D-chiro-inisitol which is associated with insulin metabolism in the brain. As with any meal plan, your personal physician should make sure it is compatible with any prescribed drugs.

The following meal plan outlines my approach to consuming foods to keep a healthy vascular system and control inflammation.

L-Lysine and Inflammation

BREAKFAST

Special attention is given to dietary fiber, probiotics and phytonutrients.

Water - Drink at least 8 ounces of filtered water. If stimulants are desired, coffee or green tea can be substituted.

Dry cereal - Use 1 cup of whole grain cereal which contains buckwheat. Add 1/4 cup of dried cranberries with soy milk to cover the cereal. Add ½ cup of active culture yogurt on top of the cereal to provide probiotics.

Supplements - Take 1 capsule of grape seed extract with resveratrol for heart health and 1 capsule of lutein and zeaxanthin for eye health. I also take 1 capsule of L-lysine to strengthen the immune system. I believe 500 mg. is satisfactory unless there are symptoms of a cold or allergy. With upper respiratory symptoms, I will take 1,000 mg. of L-lysine for a week.

At times a standard breakfast of eggs, milk and bacon can be eaten. These foods are high in L-lysine and should be eaten with as little bread as possible since bread is high in L-arginine.

This keeps the L-lysine to L-arginine ratio correct.

LUNCH

For lunch, Fast foods such as burgers, fries and carbonated beverages are rarely eaten.

Oatmeal - Use ½ cup of regular oatmeal with 1/4 cup of dried cranberries. Soy milk or almond milk is added and it is cooked in the microwave.

Water - Drink 8 ounces of filtered water.

Fruit - Fresh or frozen fruit can be added to the oatmeal or eaten separately.

Supplements - One square inch of dark chocolate is eaten for better heart health. Take 500 mg. of plant-derived vitamin C to strengthen the immune system. I take an omega-3 fish oil capsule which should contain 300 mg. each of EPA and DHA. The fish oil should be free of heavy metals and chemicals such as pesticides and antibiotics.

If oatmeal is not suitable, an active culture yogurt can be added to granola. I like the breakfast and lunch foods because they are readily available and no planning is necessary.

DINNER

The dinner meal plan uses those foods contained in an anti-inflammatory or Mediterranean meal plan. These foods come from Greece, Spain and southern Italy. Examples of these foods are olive oil, beans, whole grain cereals, fruits and vegetables combined with fish, cheese and yogurt. Mediterranean diets are found in detail with a computer search.

Attention should be paid to consuming beans, fish, cheese and yogurt to obtain the proper L-lysine to L-arginine ratio. Red meat which is high in L-lysine is not part of the Mediterranean food plan. This dinner food plan is high in phytonutrients called flavonoids. These chemicals are generally highly pigmented and strengthen the immune system. Flavonoids allow the body to utilize vitamin C more efficiently. Some of the phytonutrient rich foods are apples, blueberries, pears, grapes, blackberries, black beans, onions, mushrooms, spinach and papaya. Phytonutrients can also be found in multivitamin and mineral supplements. If there are days where pigmented foods are not in the food plan, a supplement can be taken. This type of multivitamin and mineral supplement is best when harvested from the field under organic conditions and processed immediately into tablet or capsule form to maintain the nutrients.

Approximately two times a week I make a smoothie or blended drink to replace a meal. The advantage of making a smoothie with raw fruit and vegetables is to keep the enzymes and other heat-sensitive nutrients in their most active form. Attention is made to keep calories low by not using high fructose or similar sugars. The more common foods and spices in a smoothie can be soy milk, apples, blueberries, strawberries, baby kale, grapes, bananas, avocado, protein powder, turmeric and citrus fruit.

I believe consuming all of these above foods, whether as regular food, supplements or probiotics in the proper combination, can lead to a healthier lifestyle with less disease. The next chapter will discuss other interesting aspects of our immune system and how things we do effects it.

CHAPTER 3

WORDS for COMPUTER SEARCH

D-CHIRO-INISITOL -

OMEGA-3 -

EPA (EICOSAPENTAENOIC ACID -

DHA (DOCOSAHEXAENOIC ACID -

L-Lysine and Inflammation

BUCKWHEAT -

LUTEIN -

RESVERATROL -

CHAPTER 4

Other men live to eat while I eat to live ..... Socrates

In general, things discussed in this book that I do to promote a better lifestyle should not be considered as a treatment and are not FDA approved. There are also rare toxic conditions such as hyperlysinemia and this is why your personal physician should be aware of your health care situation.

I have intentionally not listed a bibliography since all of the information included in this book can be found by computer search. If additional information is needed, I can be contacted with information listed on the page About The Author. I am very interested in the reader's experiences with L-lysine or other amino acids.

L-lysine is an essential amino acid and effects the production of collagen which is a building block of body tissues. L-lysine is also necessary for the body to produce carnitine. Carnitine is thought to facilitate fatty acid metabolism and may help with cardiovascular problems. It can be purchased as a supplement.

L-Lysine and Inflammation

Although the cause of cancer is generally not known, there have been studies on hemangiomas, cervical cancer, bladder cancer and lung cancer that uses a treatment mixture of L-lysine, L-arginine, ascorbic acid and green tea extract that appears to suppress tumor cell growth. These compounds have documented anti-inflammatory effects which may eventually help in the treatment of these types of conditions.

Herpes infections, whether oral, ocular or genital, can be treated with acyclovir type drugs either in an acute infection or in the chronic form to suppress the virus. Some patients have side effects from drug treatment. It would be interesting to study the effect foods rich in L-lysine have on the recurrence of these viral infections.

L-lysine usage has been part of many studies involving the human body. Human growth hormone production may be associated with L-lysine metabolism. L-lysine may have an anti-inflammatory effect and when combined with ascorbic acid, may decrease pain. This combination may have a beneficial effect on cardiovascular disease. L-lysine is thought to help the body absorb calcium and decrease calcium excretion. This effect on calcium along with increased collagen production may increase bone strength. These effects can be studied in detail with a computer search so each individual can decide on the validity of each claim.

Wheat flour with L-lysine added that is sent to countries with poor nutrition appears to improve that population's general health. Although there are many factors involved, the L-lysine supplementation increases the L-lysine to L-arginine ratio. This may be why the nutritional value appears to be better.

Vegans who do not eat animal protein often take L-lysine as a supplement to produce better well being. On the other hand, those who eat mostly animal protein need to add phytonutrients to their food intake to have better health.

By showing and discussing some of the possible benefits of ingesting foods high in L-lysine and low in L-arginine, I believe it gives each person the information to decide on a dietary plan that promotes better health.

CHAPTER 4

WORDS for COMPUTER SEARCH

HYPERLYSINEMIA -

CARNITINE -

ASCORBIC ACID -

GROWTH HORMONE -

Dr. Robert G. King Jr.

HEMANGIOMA -

VEGAN

CONCLUSION

To lengthen thy life, lessen thy meals .... Benjamin Franklin

As we age, our body's medical problems change. When younger, we often have acute medical problems which require short term treatments to heal the problem. In later life our medical problems often cannot be eliminated: however, they can be controlled with long-term treatments which produce satisfactory results. One example is the treatment of dry macula retinal degeneration with vitamin supplements to stabilize the retina. This satisfactory treatment leads one to question whether our nutrition in later life is sufficient to maintain our health without supplementation with vitamins, minerals, phytonutrients, probiotics and various essential amino acids. Recently, while reviewing ocular nutritional information, my interest in the amino acid L-lysine was renewed. I had prescribed the L-lysine supplement years ago to help prevent the reoccurrence of herpetic corneal infections. This anti-viral effect along with it's possible anti-inflammatory properties may make L-lysine beneficial as a supplement to strengthen our health in general.

L-Lysine and Inflammation

I have described my food plan that has the objective of ingesting nutrients to strengthen the immune system and result in a healthier life style. L-lysine is one of those nutrients I take daily.

I take 500 mg. of L-lysine daily and increase it to 1,000 mg. daily for one week if there are signs of infection such as aching or a fever.

Poor nutrition produces profound changes in our health. We believe our food intake is generally satisfactory; however, often we consume foods that are over processed, high in calories with chemical stabilizers and preservatives. This type of food slowly leads to chronic inflammation and poor health. Medications can help control these medical problems but do not correct the cause which often poor nutrition. I hope this discussion of ways to improve our nutrition and produce improved health will result in a healthier life style and increased longevity.

ABOUT THE AUTHOR

Robert G. King, Jr., M.D., graduated from the University of Virginia in 1962. He served in the Army Medical Corps from 1963 thru 1965. He completed his Ophthalmology residency at the Medical College of Virginia in 1968 and since has been in private practice. Any person who would like to contact the author concerning L-lysine and nutrition can use the address as follows:

>Robert G. King, Jr., M.D.
>2821 North Parham Road
>Henrico, Virginia 23294
>E-mail : BandBGifts@aol.com